KIRT TAYLOR

Intermittent fasting

Made simple: Lose Weight and Boost Health

This book was professionally typeset on Reedsy.
Find out more at reedsy.com

Contents

1

INTRODUCTION

Welcome to the world of Intermittent Fasting – an exhilarating journey that I am thrilled to embark upon with you in this book. If you're anything like me, you've likely explored a multitude of diets and invested in a cornucopia of weight loss supplements, unknowingly contributing to a multi-billion-dollar market. The dietary landscape can often be confusing, leaving you with minimal results or, worse, a deep-seated disdain for the process. The idea of Intermittent Fasting initially struck me as complex and somewhat daunting – the notion of abstaining from food for 16 hours felt arduous, particularly for someone who relishes their meals. I contemplated it as just another weight loss endeavor not worth pursuing. Little did I realize that Intermittent Fasting held within it a world of untapped potential.

Recently, I had the pleasure of reuniting with old friends who had undergone remarkable transformations. The gentleman had shed over 100 pounds, while the lady had lost 40, and the change in their appearances was truly astonishing. They exuded confidence, happiness, and a newfound sense of fitness. Given my history of fluctuating weight and the significant financial investments in weight loss attempts, their newfound vitality intrigued me. I couldn't help but inquire about their secret. Their response was simple yet profound – Intermittent Fasting.

Intrigued, I delved into the subject, immersing myself in articles and research, and what I discovered was far more than I'd ever expected. The benefits of Intermittent Fasting far outweighed the minor inconvenience of occasional hunger pangs. I was captivated by the concept and felt compelled to share it with anyone grappling with weight issues or health concerns. What's more, I was determined to make it easily accessible and comprehensible. You see, it doesn't have to be complicated, and in this concise book, I've distilled all the fundamental knowledge you require to thrive with Intermittent Fasting. My aim is to save you countless hours of research and make your journey to success in this program as straightforward as possible. I want you to experience the profound health, happiness, and vitality that Intermittent Fasting can bring to your life.

So, if you're reading this and feeling the spark of excitement to transform your life, then seize this opportunity and take action! Much like a car waiting for the ignition key to turn, let's turn that key to unlock a healthier, happier you.

To your health!

WHAT IS INTERMITTENT FASTING

How often have you found yourself trapped in the clutches of restrictive diets that dictate every morsel you should consume throughout the day? The relentless regimen of specific meal plans for breakfast, lunch, and dinner can be utterly exhausting, not to mention uninspiring. The concept of Intermittent Fasting offers a refreshing departure from the conventional dieting narrative. It's less about the "what" and more about the "when" – a fundamental shift in perspective.

Intermittent Fasting revolves around the cyclical pattern of eating and fasting, a concept that may be more familiar to you than you realize. Think about it: every night when you go to sleep, you unknowingly commence a fasting period. It's an inherent part of our daily rhythm. And when you awaken, your morning ritual often includes breaking the overnight fast – hence the term "breakfast."

The beauty of Intermittent Fasting lies in its simplicity. It's about harnessing the power of timing to not only enhance your health but also to achieve weight loss. To embark on this journey successfully, all you need is a well-structured game plan. A thoughtful and strategic approach to Intermittent Fasting can unlock a world of benefits. It's time to explore the various programs and methodologies that underpin this approach, as they hold the key to a healthier and leaner you. So, let's delve into the diverse fasting programs that Intermittent Fasting has to offer and tailor them to your unique goals and lifestyle.

1. 16/8 Method: This method involves fasting for 16 hours each day and restricting your eating to an 8-hour window. For example, you might eat between 12:00 PM and 8:00 PM and fast from 8:00 PM to 12:00 PM the next day.

2. 5:2 Diet: In this approach, you consume your regular diet for five days of the week and drastically reduce your calorie intake (usually around 500-600 calories) on the other two non-consecutive days.

3. Eat-Stop-Eat: This method involves fasting for a full 24 hours once or twice a week. For example, you might eat dinner at 7:00 PM and then fast until the next day's dinner at 7:00 PM.

4. Alternate-Day Fasting: With this approach, you alternate between days of regular eating and days of fasting or consuming very few calories.

5. Warrior Diet: This method involves fasting for 20 hours and eating one large meal in a 4-hour eating window, typically in the evening.

When embarking on the journey of Intermittent Fasting, you'll quickly discover a variety of fasting methods, each offering its unique appeal. It's natural to wonder which one aligns best with your lifestyle and preferences. As I mentioned earlier, I'm a firm believer in simplicity – a practical, no-nonsense approach to shedding those extra pounds. The notion of undertaking something as intense as the warrior diet didn't resonate with me, and perhaps you can relate. Instead, my journey with Intermittent Fasting steered me towards the 16/8 method, a method that not only stands out as one of the most popular but is also incredibly straightforward and easy to follow.

The 16/8 method essentially revolves around a 16-hour fasting window followed by an 8-hour eating period. As mentioned earlier, this means your last meal of the day might be around 8:00 PM, and you won't eat again until 12:00 PM the next day. No breakfast, you ask? That's correct! It might seem daunting at first, especially if you're accustomed to that morning meal, but we'll dive into the intricacies of food and eating with Intermittent Fasting in a later chapter. The initial steps of any new endeavor can indeed be a tad uncomfortable, but rest assured, your body is an incredibly adaptable marvel. It will quickly acclimate to your new routine and begin treating you like the royalty you are.

Once you break your fast at noon, you'll have a generous 8-hour window to nourish yourself. It's worth noting that the quality of fuel you choose to put into your "gas tank" – your body – will inevitably influence your energy output. I often draw a parallel to a race car: just as low-octane fuel wouldn't fuel a race car's engine as effectively as high-octane fuel would, the same applies to the foods we consume. You've got the idea, right? So, those tempting doughnuts may need to take a backseat as you navigate this journey to a healthier you.

If you like the 16/8 method you don't have to be very strict on using just the 8:00 PM - 12:00 PM time frame. If you have a hectic schedule just make up another time! Let me give you some examples.

Popular 16/8 time windows include:
   7 am to 3 pm
   9 am to 5 pm
   12 pm to 8 pm
   2 pm to 10 pm

Just pick a time and go! Most of the fasting time would be while you are sleeping. While you are in the fasting time frame, the idea is to not consume any calories. You may drink water, coffee, tea or a no-calorie beverage. Give it a shot! I believe in you!

THE 16:8 DIET

	DAY 1	DAY 2	DAY 3	DAY 4	DAY 5	DAY 6	DAY 7
MIDNIGHT 4 AM 8 AM	FAST	FAST	FAST	FAST	FAST	FAST	FAST
12 PM	First meal	First meal	First meal	First meal	First meal	First meal	First meal
4 PM	Last meal by 8PM	Last meal by 8PM	Last meal by 8PM	Last meal by 8PM	Last meal by 8PM	Last meal by 8PM	Last meal by 8PM
8 PM MIDNIGHT	FAST	FAST	FAST	FAST	FAST	FAST	FAST

3

WHAT DO YOU EAT

Isn't it funny how, when it comes to diets, you often hear the same advice reiterated in various forms? The chorus of "avoid sugars, shun carbs, steer clear of processed foods, and prioritize veggies and lean proteins" is like the greatest hits album that never goes out of style. It's true, as we discussed earlier with the race car analogy, putting high-octane fuel into your body can indeed yield impressive results. But does this mean bidding farewell to fast food or relegating cookies to the "no-go" zone? Who can resist the temptation of a piping hot fudge sundae now and then? That's where the beauty of our human bodies comes into play. They have an uncanny way of signaling what's right and what's not. How many times have you felt fantastic after munching on an apple? Now, compare that to the feeling after indulging in that delectable hot fudge sundae.

Remember, with Intermittent Fasting, it's not so much about what you eat as it is about when you eat. So, why should you care about what goes on your plate? Well, your food choices can be your ticket to achieving your goals more efficiently and unlocking maximum results. Let's dig into some of those delectable food options, which you can savor during the 8 hours of sheer gastronomic delight when you're not fasting. And remember, there's room for that occasional hot fudge sundae – life's too short not to enjoy its sweet pleasures!

Well-Balanced Meals: It's essential to strategize your meals with a keen eye on balance. Opt for well-rounded dishes that encompass a harmonious blend of carbohydrates, proteins, and healthy fats. This balanced approach isn't just about satisfying your palate; it's about fueling your body for optimal performance. Such meals provide a steady stream of energy, stave off those untimely hunger pangs, and foster a sense of fullness that complements your Intermittent Fasting journey seamlessly. The key to success in this approach lies in crafting meals that serve as a source of sustained vitality, making your fasting periods more manageable and productive.

16:8 Intermittent Fasting — 7 Day Meal Plan

	First meal: 12 PM	Snack (optional)	Last meal end time: 8 PM
DAY 1	• 2 boiled eggs • ½ avocado • Breakfast salad with leafy greens and lemon • 1 slice whole wheat bread	• 10-12 raw almonds • 2 dried figs • 1 cup green tea	• 8 tbsp. roasted vegetables • 4 tbsp. brown rice • Salad (You can add lemon, apple cider vinegar and olive oil to your salad.) 
DAY 2	Oatmeal Bowl: • 4 tbsp. oatmeal • 1 cup milk Toppings: • 1 tbsp. unsweetened peanut butter • 1 apple or 1 banana	• 1 handful pumpkin seeds • 2 dried apricots • 1 cup green tea	• 180 g grilled chicken breast • 4 tbsp. quinoa • Salad (You can add lemon, apple cider vinegar and olive oil to your salad.) 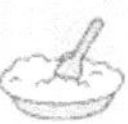
DAY 3	• Omelette with 2 eggs and cheese • Salad with leafy greens	• 1 cup coffee • 1 banana • 4-5 walnuts	• Vegetable soup • 150 g red meat • 4 tbsp. buckwheat 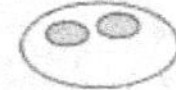
DAY 4	• 2 boiled eggs • ½ avocado • Breakfast salad with leafy greens and lemon • 1 slice whole-wheat bread	• 10 hazelnuts • 1 cup fennel tea	• Grilled salmon with potatoes • Salad 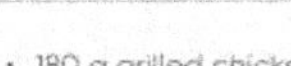
DAY 5	Oatmeal Bowl: 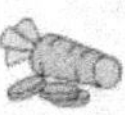 • 4 tbsp. oatmeal • 1 cup of milk Toppings: • 1 tbsp. of unsweetened peanut butter • 1 apple or 1 banana	• 1 apple • 5-6 raw cashews	• 4 meatballs (160 g total) • 4 tbsp. pasta • Salad (You can add lemon, apple cider vinegar and olive oil to your salad.)
DAY 6	• Omelette with 2 eggs and cheese • 1 slice whole wheat bread • Salad with leafy greens and carrot 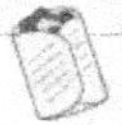	• 2 squares dark chocolate • 1 cup coffee	• 180 g grilled chicken breast • 4 tbsp. brown rice • Green salad with squeezed lemon and olive oil dressing
DAY 7	• 2 boiled eggs • ½ avocado • Breakfast salad with leafy greens and lemon • 1 slice whole wheat bread	• 10 raw almonds • 1 cup mint tea 	• 1 bowl vegetable soup • 1 plate legumes (chickpeas/lentils/beans) • Green salad with squeezed lemon and olive oil dressing

*tbsp. = tablespoon
*tsp. = teaspoon

Lean Protein Sources: A fundamental component of your well-structured meals should be lean sources of protein. These might encompass an array of options, including poultry, fish, lean cuts of meat, tofu, tempeh, beans, and legumes. Why is protein so crucial, you might ask? Well, it plays an integral role in muscle maintenance, ensuring that your body continues to function at its best. Not only that, but protein has another superpower – it's remarkably effective at promoting satiety. In other words, it helps you feel full, which can be a game-changer during your Intermittent Fasting regimen. By incorporating these lean protein sources into your meals, you'll set yourself up for a journey that's both nutritious and satisfying. Your body will thank you for it!

Incorporate Healthy Fats: When planning your meals, don't overlook the importance of integrating sources of healthy fats. This category includes nutrient-rich foods such as avocados, nuts, seeds, eggs, and olive oil. Here's a fascinating tidbit: did you know that specific vitamins, namely A, D, E, and K, require the presence of healthy fats in your body to be fully absorbed and utilized? These fats play a pivotal role in ensuring that these essential vitamins can effectively do their job. In addition to this critical function, healthy fats also provide your body with essential fatty acids, which are integral for overall well-being. Another noteworthy advantage is their contribution to a lasting sense of fullness, a factor that can be a significant asset during your Intermittent Fasting journey. By welcoming these wholesome fats into your diet, you'll be creating a foundation for meals that are not only delicious but also nutritionally sound. Your body will appreciate the nourishment!

Complex Carbohydrates: Opting for complex carbohydrates is a prudent choice in crafting your Intermittent Fasting meals. This category includes whole grains such as brown rice, quinoa, and whole wheat products. The beauty of these complex carbohydrates lies in their ability to release energy gradually, resulting in more sustained vitality throughout the day. Moreover, they contribute to stabilizing blood sugar levels, a crucial factor in maintaining overall health. By choosing complex carbohydrates for your meals, you're making a well-informed decision that aligns with your Intermittent Fasting goals. These nutrient-rich options provide not only a steady source of energy but also support the balance of blood sugar, ensuring your journey is characterized by sustained wellness and vigor. Your body will thrive on these thoughtful meal choices.

Fiber-Rich Foods: In the realm of well-rounded meal planning for your Intermittent Fasting journey, it's crucial to give a nod to foods high in fiber. This category encompasses an array of delectable options, including a colorful assortment of vegetables, a variety of fruits, whole grains, and legumes. The remarkable attribute of these fiber-rich foods is their capacity to promote both a lasting sense of fullness and optimal digestive health.

By including these nutrient-dense options in your diet, you're ensuring that your journey through Intermittent Fasting is not only satisfying but also conducive to a healthy digestive system. The fiber content in these foods not only keeps you feeling satisfied for more extended periods but also aids in regular and efficient digestion. This makes them indispensable components of your meals, ensuring that your well-being remains a top priority throughout your Intermittent Fasting experience. Your body will undoubtedly thank you for these nourishing choices!

Staying well-hydrated: A fundamental pillar of your Intermittent Fasting journey, and it can't be emphasized enough. To ensure you maintain proper hydration, make a habit of drinking an ample amount of water, herbal tea, or healthy hydration drink (sans added sugar or cream) during your designated eating windows. Hydration plays a vital role in managing hunger, which can be a game-changer during fasting periods. If plain water isn't enticing, feel free to infuse it with a twist by adding a dash of lemon, a slice of cucumber, or a few fresh mint leaves.

Another handy tip to gauge your hydration status is to observe the color of your urine. Dark or yellowish urine can signal dehydration, so it's important to address this by increasing your fluid intake. It's essential to remember that while Intermittent Fasting focuses on when you eat, maintaining proper hydration is equally critical to your success.

Keeping an eye on portion sizes during your eating windows is another wise move to prevent overeating. This ensures that you can fully savor your meals in the 8-hour window while still working toward your desired results. The key lies in finding the right balance between speed and size as you embark on your journey toward improved health and well-being.

Portion Control: As you savor your meals during your designated eating windows, exercising portion control is of paramount importance. It's easy to get carried away, especially when you're enjoying delicious whole foods. The key here is to strike a balance between delighting in your food and ensuring you don't overindulge.

Keeping an eye on portion sizes during your eating windows is another wise move to prevent overeating. This ensures that you can fully savor your meals in the 8-hour window while still working toward your desired results. The key lies in finding the right balance between speed and size as you embark on your journey toward improved health and well-being.

Whole Foods: In the realm of Intermittent Fasting, whole, unprocessed foods take center stage. These nutrient-rich options, replete with vitamins and minerals, are your allies in this journey. Whole foods include an array of choices such as fresh fruits, a diverse assortment of vegetables, whole grains, lean proteins, nuts, seeds, and wholesome potatoes.

What sets these foods apart is their richness in both protein and dietary fiber, making them champions in the realm of satiety. Their protein content helps keep those hunger pangs at bay, ensuring you're not tempted to reach for snacks in between your fasting periods. By incorporating these whole foods into your Intermittent Fasting routine, you're not only promoting fullness but also embracing a healthier and more nutritious path to your desired results. Your body will undoubtedly appreciate these nourishing choices.

Minimize Processed Foods: While Intermittent Fasting does allow for some flexibility in your food choices, it's beneficial to exercise caution when it comes to processed foods. These items, often characterized by their convenience, include snacks like crackers, pretzels, or cupcakes. While they can be incorporated into your eating windows, it's essential to be mindful of their limited nutritional value. Many processed foods lack the nutrients your body craves and may not provide the lasting fullness you desire.

Furthermore, it's advisable to steer clear of foods high in added sugars, as these can potentially disrupt your fasting goals. However, it's worth noting that special occasions, such as attending a game or a movie, can call for indulging in treats like a bag of popcorn or some junior mints. The key lies in enjoying these treats within the confines of your 8-hour eating window, ensuring that your Intermittent Fasting experience remains both enjoyable and aligned with your health objectives. Your body will thrive when it's nourished with a balance of wholesome foods.

Meal Timing: The beauty of Intermittent Fasting lies in its flexibility, allowing you to tailor your meal timing to your fasting schedule. For instance, if you're embracing the 16/8 fasting pattern, your meal timing can be a delightful and practical part of your daily routine. Imagine savoring your first meal around noon, ensuring you fuel your body for the hours ahead, and culminating your day with a satisfying last meal around 8:00 PM.

This schedule not only complements your fasting goals but also offers a sense of structure and predictability to your day. It's a delightful dance of nourishment within your chosen eating window, allowing you to make the most of your Intermittent Fasting journey. By harmonizing your meal timing with your fasting pattern, you're crafting a personalized and effective approach to health and well-being. So, go ahead, let your meal timing be a joyful part of your daily rhythm on this path to a healthier you!

That was indeed a fun journey through the world of healthy choices and Intermittent Fasting! Are you already starting to feel the positive effects of these mindful decisions? You now have a delightful 8-hour window to plan your meals and relish them with a focus on well-being.

And here's some food for thought from Johns Hopkins neuroscientist Mark Mattson, a pioneer with 25 years of experience studying intermittent fasting. He shares, "Intermittent fasting contrasts with the normal eating pattern for most Americans, who eat throughout their waking hours." Mattson's insights underscore the significance of Intermittent Fasting, especially in a culture where constant snacking and continuous eating are the norm.

The core idea behind Intermittent Fasting is to shift from running on the calories from your last meal to addressing the real challenge—burning those stored fats. Let's ignite the flames and tackle those fatty tissues head-on, maybe not with a flamethrower, but with a fierce commitment to your health and well-being!

4

FAST, EXERCISE, SLEEP

I ntermittent Fasting, often celebrated for its effectiveness in weight management, ushers in a paradigm shift in how we approach calorie consumption. Within the confines of an 8-hour eating window, a natural reduction in calorie intake occurs, laying the foundation for successful weight loss. However, it's essential to strike a balance, for excessive indulgence can counteract the method's benefits. Beyond calorie control, this dietary strategy orchestrates a symphony of metabolic changes. It adeptly lowers insulin levels and orchestrates a surge in growth hormone production—two indispensable players in regulating metabolism, catalyzing fat breakdown, and safeguarding precious muscle mass.

But here's where it gets interesting! Intermittent Fasting is not a lone warrior; it's part of a dynamic trio along with exercise and sleep. If your objective leans towards building muscle, it's important to acknowledge that this endeavor thrives on ample fuel, something that Intermittent Fasting might restrict. This dietary approach is often aligned more with weight loss than muscle gain, considering the calorie deficit it promotes. But fear not, for it still plays a vital role in your holistic weight management journey. With the addition of exercise and quality sleep, you'll witness the three working in tandem, creating a harmonious symphony of health and well-being!

The timing of your workouts in the realm of intermittent fasting is a strategic element that can influence the overall success of your fitness regimen. Consider the fasting window's duration, as seen in the 16/8 method. If this is your chosen approach, it's worth noting that incorporating exercise within your fasting period, especially in the morning, can seamlessly meld into your routine.

Some individuals even prefer working out while in a fasted state, as it may enhance the body's fat-burning mechanisms. The choice of exercise is another facet to contemplate. If weightlifting is your preferred activity, scheduling these sessions within your 8-hour eating window is highly recommended. This allows you to ingest vital post-workout nutrients, which are instrumental in facilitating muscle growth. In contrast, cardio workouts offer more flexibility, as they can be accommodated in either fasting or eating periods, catering to your personal preferences and fitness objectives. The key is to align your exercise timing with your unique goals and routines.

Hydration assumes paramount importance, especially in the context of fasting and exercise. It's crucial to maintain adequate fluid intake to support your overall well-being. As you fast, your body relies on internal fat stores for energy, and hydration becomes indispensable in this process. Therefore, during your fasting window, make it a priority to consume ample fluids. You can opt for a variety of non-caloric beverages, including water, herbal tea, and black coffee, which are permissible during fasting periods. These choices not only quench your thirst but also contribute to your body's hydration status. Proper hydration ensures that your workouts are safe and effective, as it aids in temperature regulation, circulation, and the transport of essential nutrients to your muscles. By focusing on staying well-hydrated throughout your fasting journey, you empower your body to perform optimally and enhance the benefits of both fasting and exercise.

The nature and intensity of your exercise regimen should be thoughtfully considered when incorporating it into your fasting routine. Light to moderate physical activities such as walking, yoga, or low-intensity cardio tend to be well-tolerated during fasting periods. These activities can complement your fasting journey by helping you burn calories and maintain an active lifestyle without excessive strain.

The nature and intensity of your exercise regimen should be thoughtfully considered when incorporating it into your fasting routine. Light to moderate physical activities such as walking, yoga, or low-intensity cardio tend to be well-tolerated during fasting periods. These activities can complement your fasting journey by helping you burn calories and maintain an active lifestyle without excessive strain.

However, when it comes to high-intensity workouts or heavy weightlifting, there are additional factors to contemplate, particularly if you find yourself in an extended fasting state. These types of exercise can be more demanding on the body and may require a closer look at your energy levels and nutritional requirements.

It's essential to align your exercise goals with your fasting objectives. If your primary aim is fat loss, then a combination of cardiovascular workouts and some form of resistance training is beneficial. While muscle building typically requires a surplus of calories, incorporating weightlifting, even with body weights or dumbbells, can help you maintain and preserve muscle mass during fasting. This ensures that your body continues to burn fat while optimizing your overall body composition. The key is to find the right balance between exercise intensity and fasting goals, adapting your routine to suit your individual preferences and capacity. By staying active and engaging in appropriate exercise, you not only support your fasting efforts but also promote your overall health and well-being.

Listening to your body is a fundamental principle when embarking on an intermittent fasting journey, particularly in conjunction with an exercise regimen. It's essential to recognize that responses to fasting can vary significantly from one individual to another. Paying close attention to your body's cues is paramount to ensuring a safe and effective fasting and exercise experience.While some people may find themselves energized and able to perform well during fasting periods, others might encounter sensations of fatigue or dizziness. These individual responses can be influenced by factors such as fasting duration, time of day, and the type of exercise undertaken.

Your body's signals are invaluable indicators of what's working best for you. If you feel invigorated and perform at your peak during fasting, you can optimize your exercise schedule to harness this newfound energy. However, if you experience fatigue or dizziness, it's crucial to be responsive and adaptive. You might consider shifting your workout to a different time or choosing exercises that align better with your fasting state.

In this dynamic interplay between fasting and exercise, customization based on your body's feedback is key. Your goal is to create a balanced approach that caters to your unique needs and preferences. By remaining attentive to your body's messages, you'll not only maximize the benefits of intermittent fasting but also ensure your overall well-being throughout the process.

Post-workout nutrition and sleep is a critical component of your exercise routine, regardless of whether you're incorporating intermittent fasting. This essential phase revolves around supplying your body with the necessary nutrients to support recovery and muscle repair, ensuring that your workouts yield the best possible results.

A well-balanced meal or snack following your workout should ideally include a combination of protein, carbohydrates, and healthy fats. Protein aids in muscle repair, while carbohydrates replenish glycogen stores and provide energy for your body. Healthy fats play a role in overall nutritional balance and help regulate numerous bodily functions.

The timing of this post-workout nourishment depends on your fasting schedule and individual preferences. Some individuals may choose to work out during their eating window, allowing them to have their post-workout meal or snack immediately after exercise. This approach can be particularly advantageous for muscle recovery and overall energy replenishment.

On the other hand, you might opt for fasting before your workout. In this case, it's essential to listen to your body's signals. If you feel comfortable and energized during your workout while fasting, that's perfectly acceptable. However, it's crucial to prioritize your post-workout nutrition to kick start the recovery process.

In summary, the timing of your workouts within the context of intermittent fasting can be flexible. Weightlifting is often best performed during your 8-hour eating period to facilitate the intake of post-workout nutrients. Cardio workouts, being less demanding in terms of postexercise nutrition, can be scheduled at your convenience. The key to success lies in personalizing your approach, paying attention to your body's needs, and reacting accordingly, ensuring that your fitness goals are well-supported within the framework of intermittent fasting. And remember, good sleep for 6-8 hours is important for overall health and recovery. Both nutrition and sleep significantly influence the effects of exercise and fasting.

Consulting a healthcare professional or a registered dietitian is a crucial step to ensure the safety and efficacy of your exercise routine within the framework of intermittent fasting. Given the individual variability in responses to fasting and exercise, seeking expert guidance becomes particularly important.

While the principle of listening to your body remains at the core of safe intermittent fasting, it's also essential to be prepared for unforeseen situations during your workouts. Feeling light-headed or fatigued while engaging in fasted cardio, for example, can happen to anyone. In such cases, it's wise to respond promptly and appropriately by pausing your workout and replenishing your body with nourishment and hydration until you feel sufficiently recovered to continue.

Carrying a snack in your gym bag is a practical precaution that ensures you have a quick and accessible source of energy when needed. This simple step can be a game-changer in maintaining your well-being during your exercise routine.

However, to establish a robust and well-informed foundation for your intermittent fasting and exercise journey, it's highly advisable to seek professional guidance. A healthcare professional or a registered dietitian can assess your individual health status, goals, and any specific dietary or medical considerations, offering tailored recommendations and strategies. Their expertise ensures that your approach to fasting and exercise aligns with your unique needs and maximizes both your health and fitness outcomes. In this collaborative effort, you can embark on your journey with confidence and assurance that your well-being remains a top priority.

In conclusion, weaving a solid 6-8 hours of sleep and exercise into your intermittent fasting journey is like mixing the perfect ingredients for a recipe of overall health and vitality. It's an exciting fusion that, when approached mindfully, can turbocharge the benefits of fasting. This dynamic trio opens doors to improved weight management, a supercharged metabolism, and boundless energy levels. The secret sauce? Finding your personal sweet spot by aligning the timing of your workout and a good night's rest with your fasting schedule, ensuring you keep the hydration levels up, picking an exercise intensity that suits your style, recharging with sleep, and delivering a post-workout refuel that your body deserves.

Whether your quest is to shed those extra pounds, reign in your metabolic control, recharge your brain and body, or simply boost your fitness levels, marrying exercise with sleep and intermittent fasting is a winning recipe. It's an approach that's both sustainable and effective, propelling you toward your health goals with unwavering momentum. Throughout this exhilarating journey, never forget to keep your safety at the forefront and let your body's cues be your trusty guide. The outcome? A platter of results that'll leave you wanting seconds. Bon appétit!

5

BENEFITS

There has been a lot of research that shows that Intermittent Fasting does more than just help you lose weight! But let's start there!

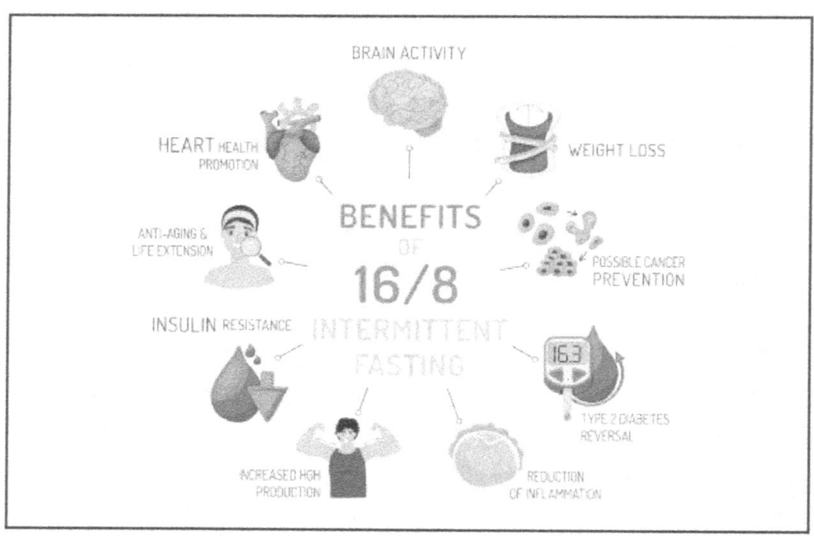

1. **Weight loss** through intermittent fasting is driven by the rhythmic cycle of eating, sleeping, and fasting, which naturally reduces calorie intake and establishes a calorie deficit, a cornerstone of successful weight management. As you embrace fasting periods, your insulin levels decline, compelling your body to tap into its fat stores for energy. This dual mechanism not only triggers fat loss but also leads to a notable reduction in overall body fat percentage. What's particularly appealing is that intermittent fasting simplifies the weight loss process, liberating you from the need for meticulous calorie counting and intricate meal preparation, making it an accessible and sustainable approach to achieving your weight loss objectives.

1. **Heart Health**: Excessive abdominal fat stands as a substantial risk factor for heart disease, making weight management crucial for reducing the risk of heart attacks. Intermittent fasting emerges as a potent ally in this endeavor, facilitating weight loss that directly contributes to heart health. Studies have underscored the benefits of fasting, revealing participants' reduction in systolic blood pressure, a critical marker of cardiovascular well-being. Moreover, intermittent fasting's potential to combat inflammation, a leading driver of heart disease and diabetes, further emphasizes its profound impact on nurturing a healthy heart.

1. **Brain Health:** The benefits of fasting on brain health exhibit variability among individuals, with some studies highlighting increased production of Brain-Derived Neurotrophic Factor (BDNF)

during fasting. BDNF is a pivotal protein that plays a vital role in fostering the maintenance and growth of nerve cells within the brain, a compelling reason to embrace fasting practices. Moreover, the capacity of fasting to reduce inflammation, both systemically and within the brain, stands as a promising strategy for averting the onset of various neurodegenerative conditions. This dual action underscores the multifaceted potential of fasting in promoting cognitive well-being.

1. **Simplicity**: The beauty of intermittent fasting lies in its ease and accessibility. There's no need to invest in special foods or follow complex dietary plans. You have the freedom to savor the foods you love within the eating time frame you personally select during your fasting period. While the journey can be further enriched by opting for whole, nourishing foods, the best part is that you're liberated from the confines of calorie counting. You hold the reins, choosing when you fast and feast, creating a schedule that suits your lifestyle. This translates to fewer meals, fewer snacks, and the delightful possibility of more time in your day to tackle those other tasks and ambitions that matter to you.

1. **Psychological Benefits**: Beyond its physical impact, intermittent fasting extends a profound influence on our mental and emotional well-being. This dietary approach becomes a pathway to discipline and self-control, granting us the power to overcome compulsive eating habits and fostering a healthier, more mindful relationship with food. The reassuring rhythm and structure of intermittent

fasting provide a refuge from the constant barrage of dietary decisions, simplifying life and instilling a comforting routine. But it doesn't stop there; this transformational journey can significantly enhance emotional well-being, offering a sanctuary where stress is diminished, leaving you with a newfound sense of calm and balance.

6

INTERMITTENT FASTING FOR WOMEN

Intermittent fasting, hailed for its numerous health advantages, has been embraced by people of all genders. Yet, women embark on a distinctive intermittent fasting journey, influenced by their remarkable hormonal and physiological makeup. This chapter delves into the captivating world of women and intermittent fasting, shedding light on the distinctive considerations and promising prospects this dietary approach offers to women.

Fasten your seat belts ladies, as we navigate the intriguing terrain of intermittent fasting tailored to your unique needs.

From hormonal intricacies to fertility concerns, we'll uncover the multifaceted dimensions of how intermittent fasting can impact women's health. Whether you're seasoned faster or just beginning to explore this path, this chapter is your compass to a healthier, more empowered you.

Hormonal Differences

In the world of intermittent fasting, women's biology sets the stage for a distinctive adventure. Their hormonal makeup, driven by the rise and fall of estrogen and progesterone during their menstrual cycles, orchestrates the intricate dance of womanhood. These hormones are not just mere players; they are conductors of the symphony that is women's health.

When women embark on the intermittent fasting journey, the fasting-induced hormonal shifts may gently ripple through the canvas of their menstrual cycles. For some, this experience may lead to changes in the regularity, duration, and intensity of their periods. The precise reasons behind these changes are still a puzzle with a few missing pieces. It is thought that fasting's influence might reach deep into the complex machinery of the hypothalamus-pituitary-gonadal axis, the regulator of the menstrual cycle.

It's essential to recognize that these effects are not universal; they vary considerably from one woman to the next. This chapter invites you to explore the tapestry of hormonal differences in the context of intermittent fasting, embracing the diversity of experiences as women navigate the fasting journey.

Fertility and Pregnancy

Women on the path to parenthood or those who find themselves expecting are walking a different journey. When considering intermittent fasting in the context of conception or pregnancy, there are unique factors at play.

Conception Concerns: For those actively trying to conceive, the fasting experience may cast ripples across the still waters of reproductive health. Fasting can affect the hormonal orchestra that regulates the menstrual cycle, potentially causing irregularities. It's an important consideration for women aiming to welcome a new life. In such cases, a more cautious approach to fasting intensity and duration is recommended. Seek the wisdom of healthcare professionals or fertility specialists to guide your path.

A Gentle Reminder for Expecting Mothers: Pregnancy is a time of profound importance, a period where two lives coexist. During this journey, fasting is generally not recommended. Why, you might ask? Because fasting can inadvertently deprive both mother and developing baby of essential nutrients. To nurture a healthy pregnancy, prioritizing a balanced diet is key. A well-rounded nutritional approach during this critical phase supports the well-being of both you and your precious cargo. Seeking the counsel of a healthcare provider ensures you're on the right track. After all, you're not alone on this incredible voyage.

Tailoring Intermittent Fasting for Women

Embracing the notion that women's responses to intermittent fasting can be wonderfully unique, it's pivotal to craft a fasting regimen that resonates with your individuality. Here are key considerations:

Fasting Flexibility: There's a rich tapestry of fasting methods to explore. The 16/8 method, fasting for 16 hours and savoring meals in an 8-hour window, often strikes a harmonious chord with women. Yet, don't hesitate to acquaint yourself with other options like the 14/10 method, which may suit those seeking to safeguard hormonal balance.

Nutrient Nurturing: When your eating window unfolds, it's the opportune time to elevate your food choices. Prioritize the richness of nutrient-dense whole foods. Fruits, vegetables, lean proteins, and whole grains should grace your plate, ensuring your body receives the bounty of essential nutrients it craves.

Body Whisperer: The language your body speaks is subtle but profoundly important. Attend to the signals it sends during fasting. Should you encounter challenges like ravenous hunger, emotional fluctuations, or hormonal intricacies, consider fine-tuning your fasting structure to restore harmony.

Healthcare Harmony: Prior to embarking on your intermittent fasting odyssey, especially if underlying health concerns are part of your story, embark on a dialogue with a healthcare provider or a registered dietitian. Their expert guidance ensures the path you choose aligns seamlessly with your well-being.

By approaching intermittent fasting as a flexible, health-focused journey, you empower yourself to harness its benefits in a manner that truly complements your unique needs and goals.

Exercise and Intermittent Fasting

Integrating exercise into your intermittent fasting journey is a treasure trove of benefits, but navigating it wisely as a woman requires attentiveness. Here's a compass to guide you:

Timing and Types: The clock ticks differently for workouts within the realm of fasting. Consider gentler, moderate exercises during fasting periods, reserving your high-octane endeavors for your eating windows.

This approach ensures that your body receives the fuel it needs at the right times.

Proper Hydration: The elixir of exercise, hydration, takes center stage when fasting. It acts as a conductor, orchestrating temperature regulation and safeguarding your overall well-being. While you sweat it out during fasting workouts, replenish with fluids like water, herbal tea, or black coffee (sans sugar or cream). These hydrating allies stand by you through thick and thin.

Body, Your Guide: Everybody is unique in its rhythm and language. Listen keenly to how yours responds. Tune in to signals of energy, fatigue, and well-being. Adjust your workout plan to reflect your body's wisdom, maintaining a balance that supports your health.

Navigating exercise and fasting as a woman requires mindful orchestration, where timing and hydration are your steady companions. The harmony between your workouts and fasting leads to a symphony of vitality and well-being.

Intermittent fasting offers women various benefits, like managing weight and improving insulin sensitivity. However, women need to understand how it might affect their hormones and consider their individual situations when embracing this diet. Whether you're looking to enhance health, lose weight, or achieve other goals, it's crucial to prioritize your well-being and consult healthcare experts when needed. Keep in mind that everyone's response to fasting is distinct, and the key to prosperous intermittent fasting for women lies in discovering the approach that suits you best.

7

CONCLUSION:EMBRACING A FASTING LIFESTYLE

As we wrap up our exhilarating journey through the world of intermittent fasting, you've uncovered the secrets of a revolutionary dietary approach that can supercharge your life. You've explored its astonishing potential to supercharge your health, achieve your weight management goals with flair, ignite your metabolic power, and perhaps even write new exciting chapters in the story of your life. In this thrilling final chapter, we're not just concluding our exploration; we're opening the door to a whole new chapter of your life, where you become the author of your health destiny. So, fasten your seat belt (pun intended), because the adventure is far from over!

1. Reflecting on Your Journey: Now, let's pause and soak in the treasure trove of wisdom you've gathered on this fasting odyssey. Intermittent fasting is more than just a mealtime makeover; it's a profound shift in how you view nourishment, a journey towards unlocking your health and wellness aspirations. It's not just about altering the clock; it's about transforming the way you see, savor, and seize life.

2. **Celebrate Your Progress**: Take a moment to revel in your victories, regardless of their size. Whether you've shed a few pounds, found newfound mental clarity, or just made those healthier choices, each step along your journey is a resounding triumph, a testament to your dedication in sculpting a healthier, more vibrant you. Celebrate the wins, no matter how small they may seem because it's these little victories that pave the way to monumental change.

3. **Adapting to Your Needs**: Recognize that intermittent fasting is a personalized journey. It's like a tailored outfit, designed to fit you, your unique lifestyle, and your preferences. Your fasting routine should be your loyal companion, adapting to your schedule, not forcing you into a rigid mold. This lifestyle is all about making it work for you, not the other way around. So, whether you prefer the 16/8 method, the 5:2 approach, or any other fasting style, make it your own, and wear it with pride. It's your fasting lifestyle, your rules!

4. **Making It Sustainable**: Think of your fasting journey as a delightful, lifelong marathon rather than a frantic sprint. The secret sauce to long-term success is sustainability. As you wholeheartedly adopt a fasting lifestyle, your main aim is to craft habits that stick with you for the long haul. It's like planting a tree that will provide shade for generations to come. So, embrace your fasting routine with joy, make it a part of your life, and let it flourish into a sustainable, lifelong habit. Because in the marathon of life, you're not just running for today; you're running for a healthier, happier, and more vibrant tomorrow.

5. **Seeking Professional Guidance**: Reaching out to healthcare professionals or registered dietitians is a wise move, especially if you have underlying health conditions or specific goals in mind. Their expert knowledge and experience can offer you invaluable guidance and

unwavering support as you navigate your fasting journey. It's like having a trustworthy compass to steer you in the right direction and ensure you reach your destination safely. So, remember that professional advice is just a consultation away, ready to empower you on your path to better health and wellness.

6. **Exploring Advanced Strategies**: With growing experience in intermittent fasting, you might develop an interest in exploring advanced fasting strategies. These can include extended fasts, where you prolong your fasting period beyond the usual daily routine, or combination approaches like the 5:2 method, which entails alternating between regular eating days and days with calorie restriction. When considering these advanced methods, it's essential to approach them mindfully, ensuring they align with your health goals, lifestyle, and comfort level. Advanced fasting techniques can introduce unique benefits, but they should be undertaken with a solid understanding of your body's needs and careful attention to your well-being.

7. **Sharing Your Success**: Share your journey! Don't keep your successes to yourself. Sharing your experiences with friends, family, and the wider community can be incredibly motivating and inspiring. Your story has the power to encourage others to embark on their own journey toward improved health and well-being. So, don't hesitate to spread the word and let your success shine as a beacon of inspiration for those around you!

8. **Embracing Balance**: Remember, intermittent fasting is just one piece of the puzzle when it comes to optimizing your health and well-being. To achieve a holistic sense of well-rounded health, don't forget to maintain a balanced approach. Incorporate regular exercise, prioritize quality sleep, and practice effective stress management as essential

components of your daily routine. By integrating these elements, you'll be on the path to achieving a vibrant and harmonious life.

Now that you've journeyed through the world of intermittent fasting, it's clear that this isn't just a diet – it's a lifestyle. It's a dynamic path to seize control of your health, enrich your connection with food, and tap into your body's remarkable ability to rebound and regenerate. The advantages of intermittent fasting transcend physical well-being and extend to sharpening mental clarity, nurturing emotional stability, and even fostering spiritual growth. This journey is about personal enhancement on diverse fronts, and you're the hero of your own story.

Embracing the fasting lifestyle is a commitment to enhancing not only your health but your entire life. As you continue to learn, adapt, and grow along this exciting journey, remember that you're on a path to lasting well-being. Whether you embarked on this journey to shed a few pounds, supercharge your energy, or simply lead a healthier life, you've uncovered a potent tool to help you achieve those goals. Intermittent fasting places the key to enduring health and vitality right in your hands. So, move forward with confidence, fully embrace the fasting lifestyle, and relish the bountiful rewards it offers. Your roa d map to wellness is now clearer than ever, and your future shines brighter than you might have imagined.

Thank you for reading this book. If you found this book helpful, I would be very appreciative if you left a favorable review for the book on Amazon!

8

RESOURCES

Intermittent Fasting: What is it, and how does it work? (2023, September 29). Johns Hopkins Medicine. https://www.hopkinsmedicine.org/health/wellness-and-prevention/intermittent-fasting-what-is-it-and-how-does-it-work

BSc, K. G. (2023, March 13). *What is intermittent fasting? Explained in human terms.* Healthline. https://www.healthline.com/nutrition/what-is-intermittent-fasting

Diet Review: Intermittent fasting for weight loss. (2022, May 17). The Nutrition Source. https://www.hsph.harvard.edu/nutritionsource/healthy-weight/diet-reviews/intermittent-fasting/

Canning, K., & Talbert, S. (2022, October 3). 6 Popular Intermittent Fasting Schedules For Weight Loss, Explained By Experts. *Women's Health.* https://www.womenshealthmag.com/weight-loss/a29349587/intermittent-fasting-schedule/

Rd, J. K. M. (2023, February 16). *9 Potential intermittent fasting side effects.*

Healthline. https://www.healthline.com/nutrition/intermittent-fasting-side-effects#5.-Fatigue-and-low-energy

Mbbs, S. M. (2021, December 21). *What happens to your body when you fast for 16 hours? 16:8 diet.* MedicineNet. https://www.medicinenet.com/what_happens_to_you_when_you_fast_for_16_hours/article.htm

Rizzo, N. (2020, September 7). *What foods are best to eat on an intermittent fasting diet?* Greatist. https://greatist.com/eat/what-to-eat-on-an-intermittent-fasting-diet#foods-to-eat-on-if

M8csanchez. (2023, February 23). *6 Things to Know About Intermittent Fasting & Working Out.* Atkins. https://www.atkins.com/how-it-works/library/articles/6-things-to-know-about-intermittent-fasting-and-working-out

CSCS, A. H., & Ritchey, C. (2023, September 22). What to know about intermittent fasting and your workouts. *Men's Health.* https://www.menshealth.com/fitness/a30300614/intermittent-fasting-working-out/

BSc, K. G. (2023b, August 29). *Intermittent Fasting 101 — The Ultimate Beginner's Guide.* Healthline. https://www.healthline.com/nutrition/intermittent-fasting-guide#weight-loss

BSc, K. G. (2021, May 13). *10 Evidence-Based Health Benefits of intermittent fasting.* Healthline. https://www.healthline.com/nutrition/10-health-benefits-of-intermittent-fasting#TOC_TITLE_HDR%20_6

Persensky, M. (2023, July 17). How intermittent fasting affects women.

Cleveland Clinic. https://health.clevelandclinic.org/intermittent-fasti ng-for-women/

Ldn, L. Y. M. R. (2023, August 8). *What you need to know about intermittent fasting for women.* EatingWell. https://www.eatingwell.com/article/ 7874733/intermittent-fasting-for-women/